HEADLINES!™

SWINE FLU

SARAH K. TASIAN, MD

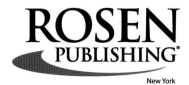

ROSEN
PUBLISHING®

New York

For Dominic Souren Tasian

Published in 2011 by The Rosen Publishing Group, Inc.
29 East 21st Street, New York, NY 10010

First Edition

Library of Congress Cataloging-in-Publication Data

Tasian, Sarah K.
Swine flu/Sarah K. Tasian. — 1st ed.
    p. cm. — (Headlines!)
Includes bibliographical references and index.
ISBN 978-1-4488-1292-9 (lib. bdg.)
1. H1N1 influenza—Popular works. 2. H1N1 influenza—United States—Popular works. I. Title.
RA644.I6T37 2011
614.5'18—dc22

2010027070

Manufactured in Malaysia

CPSIA Compliance Information: Batch #W11YA: For further information, contact Rosen Publishing, New York, New York, at 1-800-237-9932.

On the cover: A child receives the H1N1 vaccine in Miami, Florida, during the 2009 pandemic.

CONTENTS

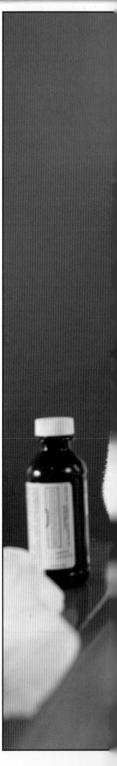

A choo! Every child and teen gets several colds or bouts of the flu each year and probably doesn't think much about them. It is annoying to have a runny or stuffy nose, cough, or sore throat, but most people feel better after a few days of rest and drinking plenty of fluids. While most of these illnesses are mild and short-lived, some last longer and can be serious, even deadly. Indeed, in 2009, a new strain of the influenza A virus called H1N1 appeared on the world scene. It quickly claimed many lives, causing international panic. This virus was dubbed the swine flu due to concerns that the strain infecting humans had originally been found in pigs.

No one knows exactly where the H1N1 virus started, but it quickly established itself as a serious infection. The virus caused many people to fall ill and resulted in thousands of deaths throughout the world. The first cases of swine flu were identified in March 2009. However, the H1N1 virus had likely infected hundreds of people during the several months before the outbreak was officially recognized.

As H1N1 spread from country to country, panic about the virus began to mount. Restrictions on airline travel were enacted. Some travelers from affected areas were quarantined for weeks or even forbidden from entering other countries.

Runny nose, cough, and fever are common symptoms of H1N1 influenza.

BREAKING NEWS • BREAKING NEWS • BREAKING NEWS • BREAKING NEWS • B
BREAKING NEWS • BREAKING NEWS • BREAKING NEWS • BREAKING NEWS • B

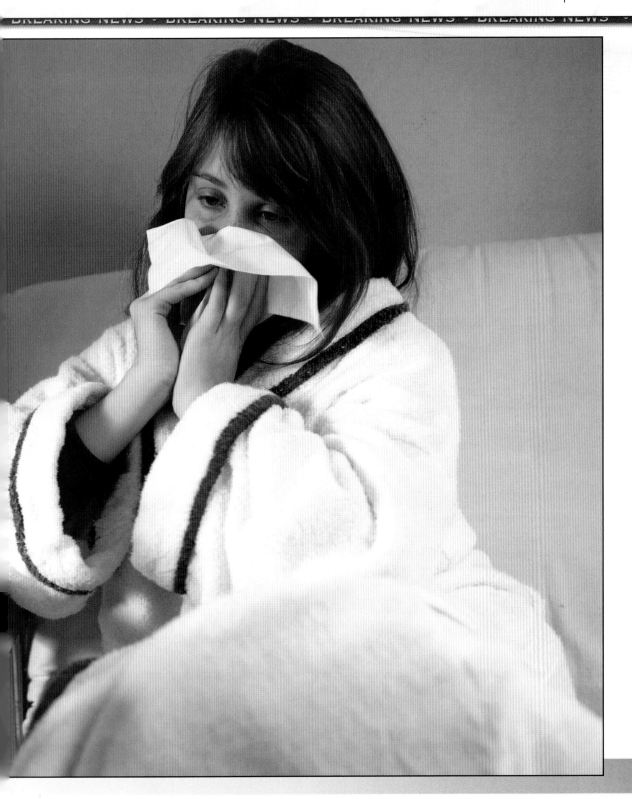

Schools and government offices in some countries were closed for months in an effort to stop the spread of this deadly virus. Despite these precautions, the swine flu pandemic continued to escalate. People in virtually every country in the world were soon affected. Even worse, there were significant delays in manufacturing the protective H1N1 vaccine, which only added to the global hysteria.

This book describes the swine flu pandemic of 2009 and its impact on global health, travel, and politics. It explores the issues surrounding the H1N1 vaccine and the impact of the vaccine shortage during the peak of the pandemic. Finally, the book describes the current state of the H1N1 virus and its potential future impact throughout the world.

CHAPTER 1

AN INTERNATIONAL EMERGENCY: THE H1N1 PANDEMIC

In the spring of 2009, it quickly became apparent that the H1N1 virus was much more severe than many other viruses. How could so many deaths and so much panic result from what seemed like a simple, common infection? To understand the swine flu pandemic of 2009, it is important to have basic knowledge of the cause of swine flu.

A NEW FLU VIRUS

Swine flu is a disease caused by a virus. Viruses are infectious particles that are not really alive; they need to enter living cells to reproduce. They infect cells and take over their internal machinery to make more virus particles. Specifically, swine flu is an infection with a type of influenza A virus called H1N1.

Viruses contain pieces of genetic material, either DNA or RNA, within a protein coat called a capsid. Some viruses also have an outer coating called an envelope, which is made up of lipids (a kind of fat) and proteins. This outer layer of proteins helps viruses attach to living cells so that they can enter and take over the cells' internal machinery. Viruses are classified or named by the kind of genetic material (DNA or RNA) they contain and the proteins in their outer coats. The virus

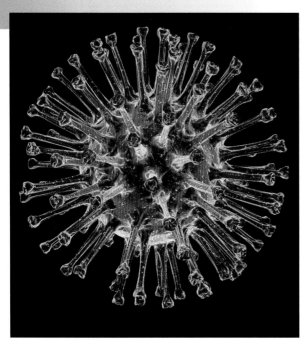

The H1N1 influenza virus has a lipid envelope with two main proteins, hemagglutinin and neuraminidase, that allow the virus to infect host cells.

that causes swine flu is named H1N1 due to the proteins hemagglutinin 1 and neuraminidase 1, which are found in its outer coating.

There are dozens of respiratory viruses that can cause the milder common cold, which tends to get better on its own in a few days. All of these cold viruses are highly contagious. They can be spread by coughing and sneezing (aerosol transmission) and by surfaces or touching (contact transmission). While common cold viruses usually cause mild illnesses, other respiratory viruses such as influenza can cause more significant symptoms. The influenza virus can cause high fever, body aches, vomiting, mental confusion, and breathing problems.

Infection with influenza, also known as the flu, may seem like no big deal. A lot of people get the flu every year, usually in the winter from about October to March. Most people get through it without a problem. However, the flu can be deadly, particularly for vulnerable groups of people such as babies, the elderly, and those with chronic health problems like diabetes. According to the Centers for Disease Control and Prevention (CDC), up to 20 percent of all people in the

United States get influenza infections every year. More than two hundred thousand people are hospitalized due to complications from the flu. Even scarier, at least thirty-six thousand deaths due to influenza are reported each year on average.

Those are the facts for the "regular" kind of flu, but the early numbers were just as frightening for the 2009 swine flu. The CDC estimated that H1N1 claimed more than seventeen thousand lives in the short time between April 2009 and mid-January 2010. Moreover, that number might have underestimated the true number of H1N1-associated deaths. (Figuring out exactly how many cases of H1N1 had occurred was tricky. Not everyone sought medical attention for symptoms, and not everyone who had medical attention was officially tested for H1N1.)

Further, the CDC called H1N1 "unusually virulent," meaning that it was a stronger strain of influenza than is commonly seen. According to the World Health Organization (WHO), a surprisingly large number of H1N1 cases occurred in healthy young people who would not typically experience such severe symptoms with the regular winter flu. The most severely affected people had to be hospitalized and even admitted to an intensive care unit (ICU) for emergency breathing assistance and other medical care. H1N1 was particularly dangerous for pregnant women. There were dozens of reports of pregnant women in the United States who required breathing tubes and mechanical ventilation (machine-supported breathing) due to the severity of their symptoms. The CDC and the Public Health Agency of Canada cautioned that anyone with severe trouble breathing, extreme vomiting, or mental confusion had to be immediately evaluated in an emergency room.

By June 2009, the WHO and CDC had declared the H1N1 outbreak a pandemic because of the widespread nature of this virus: it was affecting people throughout the world.

The H1N1 Pandemic: How Did It Begin?

Around February 2009, something strange started happening. Thousands of people in Mexico were noted to be getting very sick with high fever, runny nose, cough, extreme fatigue, and breathing trouble. Reports of similar illnesses cropped up in various countries around the world, such as New Zealand and Egypt. People's symptoms looked like those of the influenza virus. However, it was very late in the season when the flu would normally occur.

Indeed, testing these people revealed that they did have the flu, but it was a flu that had rarely been seen before. Édgar Enrique Hernández, a four-year-old boy in La Gloria, Mexico, became sick in late March 2010. Special medical testing performed on Édgar's nasal mucus revealed that he had a new form of influenza that was a mix of human, pig, and bird subtypes. This influenza was the H1N1 strain. It likely resulted from various influenza viruses mutating over time until they formed a particularly aggressive type of the virus. Édgar quickly made international news as the first laboratory-tested case of this strange new type of flu.

H1N1 had been detected previously in pigs in the United States, Canada, Argentina, Northern Ireland, and Norway, but it had never before been seen in people. As a result, health officials believed that H1N1 had been transmitted to humans from pigs. However, it was hard to know exactly when this jump between pigs and people may have occurred.

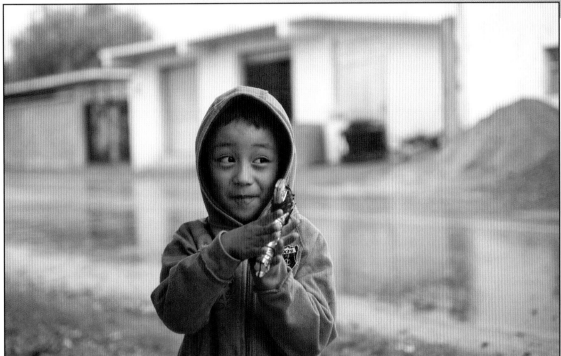

BREAKING NEWS • BREAKING NEWS • BREAKING NEWS • BREAKING NEWS • BREAKING NEWS • BREAKING

Édgar Enrique Hernández from La Gloria, Mexico, was one of the first patients with laboratory-confirmed H1N1 influenza.

Some countries feared that people were contracting H1N1 by eating infected pig products, like pork. The U.S. secretary of agriculture published a statement, which said that this idea was not correct. Some countries, like Egypt, slaughtered hundreds of thousands of pigs because of these fears, though. According to an article by Laurie Garrett in *Newsweek*, many people in La Gloria believed residents initially caught H1N1 due to poor sanitation conditions. Residents said their water supply could have been contaminated by infected waste from nearby pig farms. No pigs near La Gloria ever tested positive for H1N1, however, according to Mexico's Department of Agriculture.

H1N1: The Global Spread

H1N1 likely spread throughout the world quickly for several reasons. First, most people with swine flu did not immediately know that they were infected. People with swine flu typically do not have symptoms like runny nose or cough for twenty-four to forty-eight hours. People are highly contagious during those first few days, though. During the pandemic, many people could easily have transmitted the virus to others before they felt sick.

People are also very mobile in the twenty-first century. Travelers can take a bus, train, ship, or plane to get to almost anywhere in the world. How many times have you sat next to someone who was coughing and sneezing on a bus or plane? Trips can be long, and passengers sit close together and breathe recycled air. It is easy to imagine how a viral infection like swine flu could be passed quickly from passenger to passenger.

According to an article on the Web site Science Daily (http://www.sciencedaily.com), "Viruses love plane travel. They get to fly around the world inside a closed container while their infected carrier breathes and coughs, spreading pathogens to other passengers, either by direct contact or through the air. And once people deplane, the virus can spread to other geographical areas." The ease of national and international travel was a significant factor in how quickly H1N1 moved throughout the world.

Thousands of other cases of H1N1 were quickly diagnosed after the first one. The majority of them were in Mexico's capital, Mexico City. Cases quickly began cropping up in California and Texas, and then others were reported throughout the world. How did H1N1 spread so quickly from the small rural town of La Gloria throughout Mexico and beyond? According to Mexican officials, many people from the area of La Gloria worked in Mexico City. They likely passed on the highly contagious virus to others. People with H1N1 traveling on buses and airplanes added to the problem.

The Mexican government quickly shut down public gathering places, like schools, churches, and businesses, but it was too late. H1N1 outbreaks quickly spread throughout the world, most likely aided by the ease of international travel. Within a few short months, many thousands had been affected by this virulent strain of influenza, and hundreds were dead.

Although the first case of H1N1 was confirmed in Mexico in little Édgar Enrique Hernández, it is not known where it actually started. It could have been anywhere in the world. Some experts believe the virus gained the ability to infect humans in 2008 before the initial 2009 outbreak. One thing was certain: once able to infect people, H1N1 spread like wildfire.

OTHER INFLUENZA PANDEMICS IN RECENT HISTORY

Throughout history, viruses have mutated and caused major infections around the world, killing hundreds of thousands, even millions, of people. These widespread infections have been called epidemics (from the Greek meaning "upon people") or pandemics (from the Greek meaning "all people").

One of the most terrible pandemics in history started in 1918. It was also due to an H1N1 strain of influenza A. However, it was a different H1N1 strain than the one that caused the 2009 pandemic. The virus was known as the Spanish flu, even though it may have started somewhere other than Spain. From 1918 to 1920, it affected about five hundred million people throughout the world and resulted in at least fifty million deaths.

The Spanish flu pandemic was truly global. It quickly spread from Europe to other parts of the world, even to remote Pacific islands and far north into the Arctic. It affected not only the very young and very old, but also teens and young adults. More than half of the people who died of the Spanish flu were between twenty and forty years old, which was unusual for influenza-associated deaths.

The Spanish flu caused more deaths than World War I, which took place between 1914 and 1918, just before the pandemic. The CDC thought the crowded living conditions of World War I soldiers, poor nutrition, and improved transportation systems greatly increased the spread of the Spanish flu and its worldwide death toll. The Spanish flu is still considered the worst influenza pandemic to date.

The Asian flu pandemic occurred from 1956 to 1958. This flu was a strain of influenza A named H2N2. (It was made up of different hemagglutinin and neuraminidase than the H1N1 strains.) It is not known how many people in the world were affected, but the WHO estimates that about two million people died from the Asian flu in that short time period.

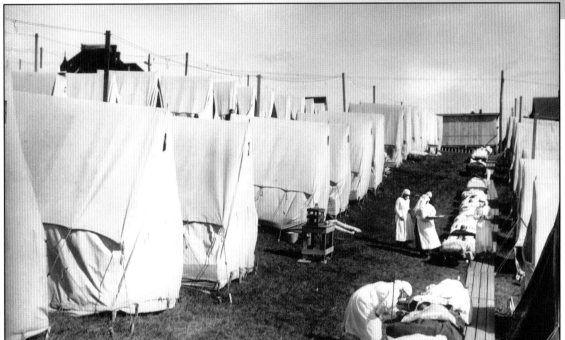

Nurses in Massachusetts care for people with influenza during the Spanish flu epidemic of 1918. Tents housed an excess of patients and separated them from others.

The Hong Kong flu pandemic lasted from 1968 to 1969 and was an H3N2 strain of influenza A. Approximately one million deaths from the Hong Kong flu have been estimated by the WHO. There have been a few other influenza epidemics during the past few decades, but none as serious as the H1N1 pandemic of 2009.

According to the CDC, influenza pandemics can occur whenever a new strain of flu emerges for which people do not have good immune system responses. Most infectious disease experts believe another influenza pandemic will occur in the future. However, it is impossible to predict which type of influenza it will be, when it will happen, or how serious it will be.

CHAPTER 2

THE PUBLIC REACTION TO H1N1

News of the unusual strength of the H1N1 virus and the rapidly increasing death toll quickly swept the world. In early spring 2009, many deaths were reported in Mexico, and some severe cases of H1N1 were cropping up in the United States. As a result, people focused their blame on Mexico. This blame was not really fair, since no one knew exactly where H1N1 had started.

FEAR SPREADS ALONG WITH THE VIRUS

Health-focused organizations like the WHO and the CDC urged people not to panic, to little effect. People throughout the world were terrified of H1N1. In many cities, it was not uncommon to see people wearing surgical face masks to protect themselves from the virus. In an effort to keep H1N1 from spreading so rapidly, government officials closed all public schools and canceled many public events in Mexico City. Many schools and businesses in the country would be closed for months.

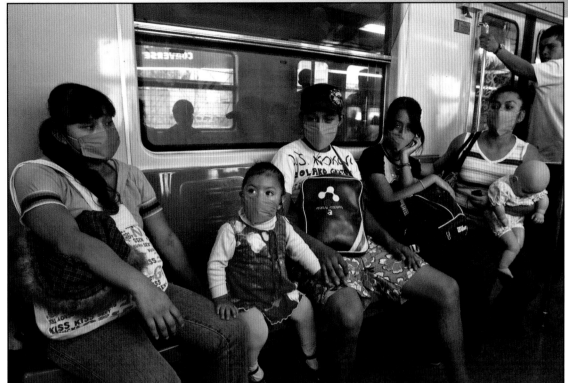

Passengers aboard a Mexican subway wear face masks to limit the spread of H1N1.

Limitations were also set on travel. According to an article in *Time* in April 2009, the U.S. Department of Homeland Security (DHS) started screening people who were traveling from countries with documented cases of H1N1. Passengers were questioned about possible flu symptoms, and anyone who was ill could be stopped from entering the country. When H1N1 was detected in Spain in May 2009, the European Union (EU) health commissioner encouraged Europeans not to travel to the United States and Mexico unless their trips were absolutely required. By October 2009, U.S. President Barack Obama had declared the swine flu a national emergency.

The Public Health Response

In the spring of 2009, hundreds of cases of H1N1 were confirmed in New York City students. In May, an international meeting was held at the New York Academy of Sciences. Experts in public health, vaccine development, and government policy gathered to discuss the swine flu pandemic and decide what to do next. Officials from the CDC and the New York City Department of Health developed national and international strategies to handle the outbreak. Vaccine developers discussed how to make a large number of H1N1 vaccines in a short period of time. Scientists from pharmaceutical companies and government laboratories talked about medicines to treat or limit the spread of H1N1.

At the meeting, Dr. Michael Shaw from the CDC said the United States was ready and had the resources to tackle the emergency. Within a month of the initial swine flu outbreak, the CDC had gathered more than two thousand respiratory samples from people to test for H1N1. With the help of state laboratories across the United States, the CDC was quickly able to identify the particular strain of influenza causing the swine flu. It was also able to test several antiviral medicines on the H1N1 strain to determine which medications would work and which would not.

Scientists at the CDC learned that the H1N1 strain was resistant to the drugs amantadine and rimantadine. This meant that these medicines were not useful in treating H1N1. On the other hand, H1N1 seemed susceptible to, or could be treated with, medicines called oseltamivir (Tamiflu) and zanamivir (Relenza). These observations

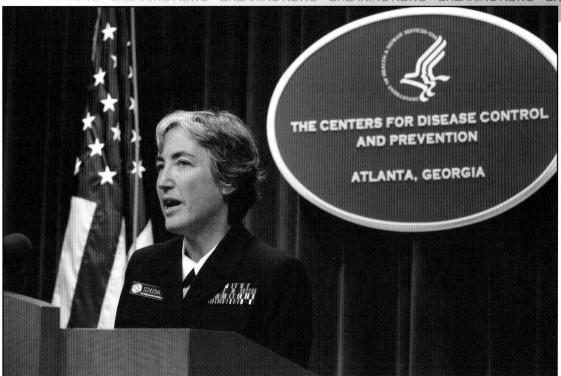

Dr. Anne Schuchat from the Centers for Disease Control and Prevention discusses the H1N1 pandemic at a press briefing in Atlanta, Georgia.

were extremely important, enabling doctors to give the right medicine to people with severe cases of swine flu. However, the information had the potential to create a national shortage of these drugs, as unaffected people quickly began asking their doctors for prescriptions for these medicines "just in case." A national shortage of the antibiotic ciprofloxacin occurred during the 2001–2002 anthrax scare when Americans began hoarding the medicine unnecessarily.

There was still a lot of work to be done. The CDC had to distribute millions of doses of antiviral medicines to treat H1N1 in very ill

PANDEMIC PREPAREDNESS

Experts at the May 2009 New York Academy of Sciences meeting emphasized the importance of emergency preparedness. By this they meant being ready at a moment's notice to tackle a major problem such as the swine flu. To help people handle the H1N1 pandemic successfully, researchers and health officials shared some of the lessons they had learned so far. They recommended the following strategies for government health officials and agencies:

• Learn everything possible about H1N1. The strain appeared seemingly out of nowhere, and public health officials had a lot to learn about the virus and how it had spread. Understanding the basic facts was critical to preparing the proper public health response to H1N1.

• Communicate and share information. The H1N1 strain was identified quickly due to labs in the United States and other countries helping each other and sharing the scientific workload.

• Practice emergency drills. The CDC was ready to mount its response rapidly because it had prepared for such a situation many times. For example, it had plans in place for quickly gathering trained emergency personnel, arranging for transportation to clinics and hospitals, and obtaining sufficient medical supplies.

patients. The CDC further had to help coordinate the development of mass production of H1N1 vaccines by several pharmaceutical companies throughout the world.

These emergency measures continued for many months as the CDC, the WHO, the Public Health Agency of Canada, and other worldwide health agencies continued to handle the H1N1 outbreak and the many problems that arose because of the pandemic.

The American Public's Fear

Despite the best efforts of national and international health organizations, public hysteria in the United States continued as more cases of H1N1 and more deaths were reported. By mid-December 2009, the CDC estimated that forty to eighty million cases of H1N1 had occurred in the United States. Of those, at least 250,000 people had required hospitalization. As of January 2010, nearly 14,300 people had died.

The Harvard School of Public Health published multiple surveys from May 2009 to February 2010 that explored the American public's opinions about the swine flu outbreak. In May 2009, one poll found that 46 percent of people were worried that they or their family members would catch H1N1 during the next year. More than half of the people surveyed noted that they were washing their hands more frequently. One-quarter reported that they were avoiding crowded public places, like shopping malls and sports arenas, to avoid catching H1N1. Eighty-three percent of people knew that H1N1 was transmitted through close contact with others with swine flu. Interestingly, though,

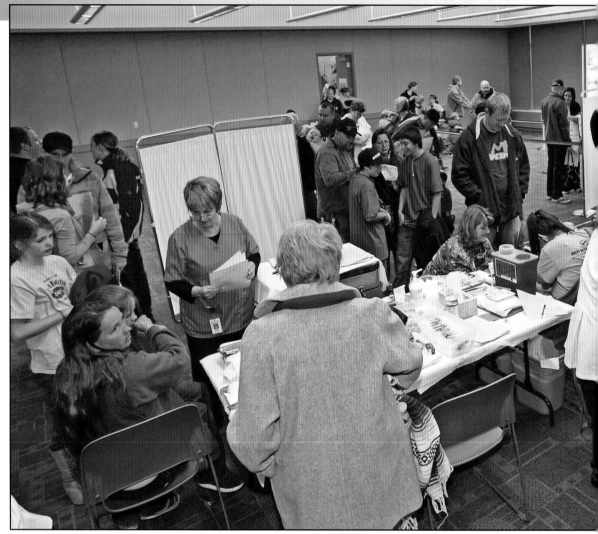

13 percent of people inaccurately thought they could catch H1N1 by eating meat from infected pigs, such as pork or bacon. Another 34 percent wrongly thought they could catch H1N1 just by being around pigs.

When there were delays in obtaining enough H1N1 vaccine in the fall of 2009, the public unease worsened. Only a small fraction of the vaccine needed was available in October 2009. The amount was far

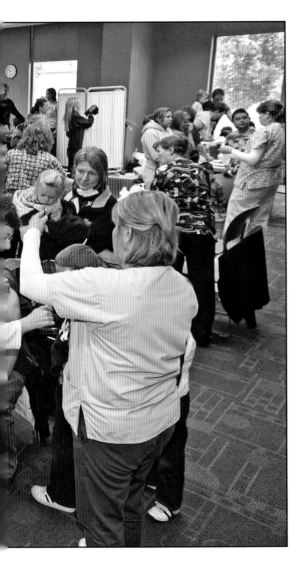

People wait patiently to receive the H1N1 influenza vaccine at a public health center in Utah.

less than what had been predicted to be available at that time. In a survey by the Harvard School of Public Health in November 2009, 70 percent of adults reported being unable to obtain the vaccine for themselves. Sixty-six percent had been unable to get the vaccine for their children. In the same survey, 82 percent of Americans recognized the lack of an adequate vaccine supply, and 41 percent called the shortage "a major problem."

As time passed, though, public fear lessened. Although the total number of cases of H1N1 was still increasing throughout the world, people seemed less afraid of the swine flu. Was this phenomenon due to better public education about and awareness of H1N1? Were people paying more attention to hygiene and staying home when they were sick to minimize spreading the illness to others? Were people less afraid because of improved vaccine availability as the H1N1 season continued? Or were people merely becoming complacent, or unconcerned?

The lessening public concern was likely a combination of all the above. The Harvard polls reported that public fear in the United States about H1N1 peaked in September 2009, with 52 percent of adults worried that they would get the swine flu. However, their worries had dramatically decreased by February 2010. At that time, 44 percent of Americans believed the swine flu "outbreak was over," and 70 percent of them thought there was an adequate H1N1 vaccine supply in their communities. Additionally, by early 2010, more than 50 percent of parents surveyed reported that they had vaccinated their children against H1N1.

Some parents chose not to get the H1N1 vaccine for their children. The most commonly reported reason for this decision was concern about the safety of the vaccine. Many parents who decided not to vaccinate stated that they could treat H1N1 with medication if their children caught the infection. Also, many did not consider the H1N1 outbreak to be as serious as public health officials once thought it was.

CHAPTER 3

H1N1 VACCINE SUPPLY AND DEMAND

With the recognition of the H1N1 pandemic, development of effective vaccines for swine flu quickly became an international priority. Because H1N1 was a new strain of influenza and because it occurred after the traditional flu season, effective vaccines did not exist immediately. The regular influenza vaccine for the 2008–2009 season was not effective against the H1N1 strain. It took months to create and mass-produce the vaccine for H1N1. The delay caused additional fear and much frustration.

VACCINE SHORTAGES

H1N1 was spreading like wildfire throughout the world in the late spring and summer of 2009. People in the United States kept hearing about the H1N1 vaccine that was coming, but weeks and months went by without any vaccine becoming available. People were panicking: how were they supposed to protect themselves and their families if there was no vaccine?

In July 2009, President Obama's administration predicted that 80 to 120 million doses of the H1N1 vaccine would be available by

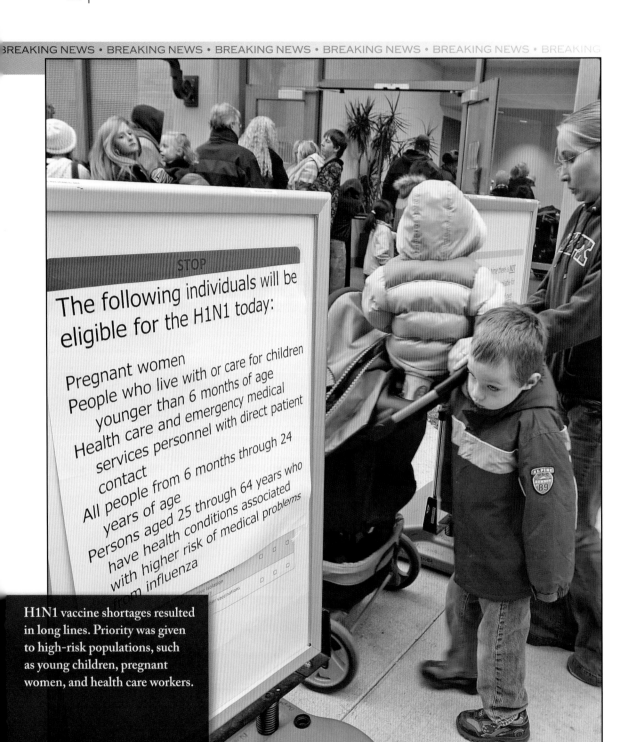

STOP

The following individuals will be eligible for the H1N1 today:

Pregnant women

People who live with or care for children younger than 6 months of age

Health care and emergency medical services personnel with direct patient contact

All people from 6 months through 24 years of age

Persons aged 25 through 64 years who have health conditions associated with higher risk of medical problems from influenza

H1N1 vaccine shortages resulted in long lines. Priority was given to high-risk populations, such as young children, pregnant women, and health care workers.

mid-October. This amount of vaccine would be enough to distribute to high-risk populations first. Additional vaccine would then be available to give to the rest of the country. The Public Health Agency of Canada planned to purchase 50.4 million doses of the vaccine on behalf of its provinces.

Five pharmaceutical companies were in charge of making the vaccine: Sanofi-Aventis, Novartis, CSL Australia, GlaxoSmithKline, and MedImmune. It was no small task. The U.S. government promised to spend more than $2 billion to buy 250 million vaccine doses. This would be enough to immunize every person in the United States who was old enough to receive the vaccine. Yet only 16.5 million doses of the H1N1 vaccine had been produced by late October 2009— about 20 percent of what had been predicted to be available. What happened?

According to a report in the *Washington Post*, Secretary of Health and Human Services Kathleen Sebelius noted that it was taking much longer than expected for the companies to make the vaccine. The companies had to grow a large amount of the H1N1 strain to make the vaccine, and the virus was not growing as quickly or as powerfully as they had predicted. In an interview with National Public Radio (NPR), Dr. Anne Schuchat, chief of the CDC's Center for Immunization and Respiratory Diseases, stated that the pharmaceutical companies had not realized they were not making enough vaccine until October. After growing the H1N1 virus, they had to test the potency, or strength, of the virus they had grown. The virus was not as potent as the companies had originally thought it would be. Therefore, they had to grow more of the virus to make the same amount of vaccine. Furthermore, there were

UNEQUAL DISTRIBUTION

According to an October 2009 article by Rebecca Ruiz in *Forbes*, having access to the H1N1 vaccine depended somewhat on geography. Although the vaccine should have been distributed based on population numbers, states were given varying amounts of the H1N1 vaccine. Florida had received the fewest vaccines—only forty-one doses for every one thousand people living in the state. Alaska, on the other hand, had received eighty-five doses per one thousand people. These discrepancies were largely attributed to differences in states' emergency preparedness.

Other disparities in distribution occurred as well. For instance, according to an article in the *San Francisco Chronicle*, several children's hospitals in California endured great delays in obtaining the H1N1 vaccine, whereas the Kaiser Permanente Group, California's largest health care provider, received the first large shipments of the vaccine. The lack of H1N1 vaccine for children at pediatric hospitals seemed unjust, and much outrage ensued in California. Public health officials noted, however, that Kaiser Permanente received the H1N1 vaccines first because the organization would be able to vaccinate large numbers of people quickly. Despite this strategy, though, thousands of high-risk patients in California had to wait several weeks to get the vaccine. Additionally, in New York City several large corporations, such as Goldman Sachs, quickly received hundreds of doses of vaccine for their employees. Many doctors' offices and hospitals had received none. This perceived inequity sparked a public outcry. Such corporations did note that early doses of vaccine were designated for their high-risk employees, such as pregnant women. In addition, many of these businesses turned over their vaccine doses to local hospitals during the peak of the vaccine shortage.

malfunctions with the machines that packaged the vaccine into vials. All of these delays and problems contributed to a serious vaccine shortage across the United States and the world.

Government officials and the American public were bewildered and angry. The WHO and the CDC had declared H1N1 an international emergency in May 2009. People had been promised that enough vaccine would be available by the early fall of 2009. The vaccine shortage left doctors' offices scrambling. Doctors had to decide who should receive the limited number of vaccines that had been distributed and stick to those tough decisions. The CDC had prioritized vaccines to be given to high-risk populations first and then to lower-risk groups. Such high-risk people included pregnant women, children and young adults, seniors, health care workers, and people with chronic health problems. Parents of infants too young to get the vaccine were also included.

Across the country, people waited for hours at clinics and pharmacies to receive the H1N1 vaccine, only to be told that there was not enough to go around. For a while, only people who were considered extremely high-risk among those special populations, such as pregnant women and children ages six months to three years, could receive the limited supply of H1N1 vaccine. Hundreds of clinics set up specifically to administer the vaccine had to be closed because there simply wasn't enough vaccine to be administered.

Meanwhile, H1N1 infection was growing to epidemic proportions across the United States. The American Medical Association (AMA) reported that H1N1 cases had been reported in forty-six states as of October 17, 2009. Shortly thereafter, President Obama declared swine flu a national emergency due to the widespread effects

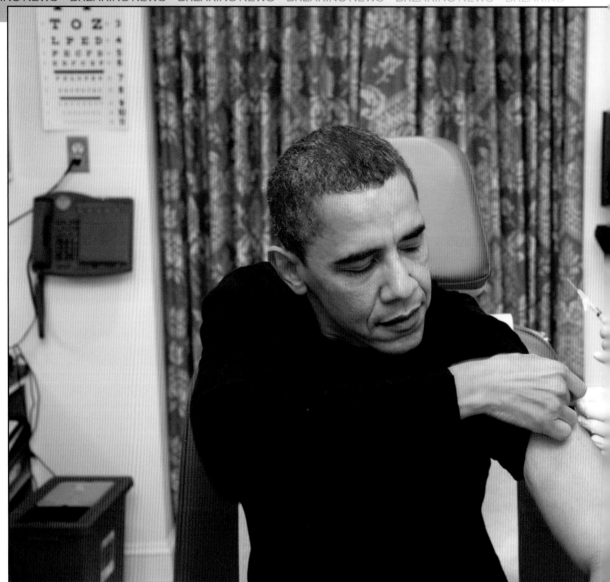

of the H1N1 virus and the vaccine shortages. By early November 2009, only 32.3 million doses of the vaccine were available. According to officials at the U.S. Department of Health and Human Services (HHS), it was impossible to predict when an adequate supply would

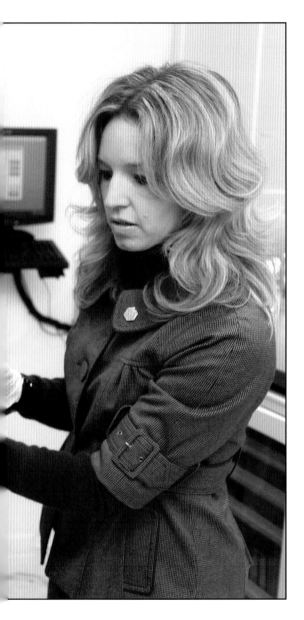

President Barack Obama rolls up his sleeve to receive the H1N1 influenza vaccine.

be ready. Furthermore, another wave of H1N1 infection had been predicted for November or December 2009. People began to worry that by the time enough H1N1 vaccine was available, it would be too late in the swine flu season for it to be effective. It takes about three or four weeks for the body to make sufficient protective antibodies in response to vaccination, and H1N1 had already infected tens of thousands of people throughout the country.

Vaccine Safety Concerns

Many parents were worried about the safety of the H1N1 vaccine for themselves and their children. They were concerned that the new vaccine might have unknown side effects. Despite the CDC's recommendation that the H1N1 vaccine was the

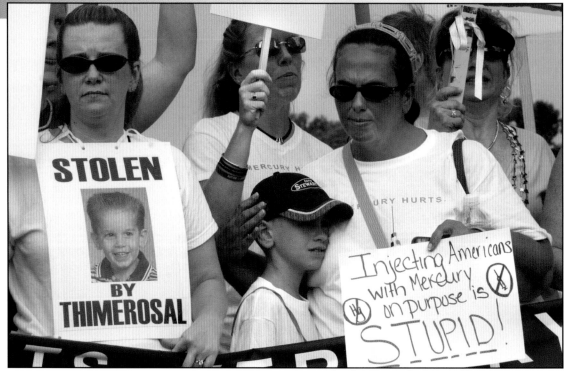

Demonstrators protest the use of thimerosal (a mercury-based preservative) in vaccines. No definitive link between diseases of the nervous system and thimerosal has been proved.

best way to prevent infection, many Americans chose not to get vaccinated. High-profile political commentators, such as conservative radio host Rush Limbaugh and liberal comedian Bill Maher, promoted skepticism about H1N1 immunization. Were people's fears grounded in reality?

Some Americans expressed concern that the H1N1 vaccine would contain the chemical thimerosal, which is derived from mercury. They feared that the chemical caused birth defects. However, the CDC has found no proven link between thimerosal and birth defects. Further, the H1N1 vaccine was being made thimerosal-free to be given to pregnant women. People also worried that because the H1N1 vaccine had never been used before, they would be guinea pigs for an untested vaccine. In reality, the H1N1 vaccine was created with similar methods and components used to make the seasonal flu vaccine. Millions of Americans and Canadians safely receive these flu shots each year.

After it was distributed, a small number of harmful side effects from the H1N1 vaccine were reported. However, a review by the National Institutes of Health (NIH) concluded that the H1N1 vaccine's safety profile is similar to that of the seasonal flu vaccine.

CHAPTER 4

PREVENTING AND TREATING SWINE FLU: HOW TO KEEP YOURSELF HEALTHY

U nfortunately, there are no guaranteed ways of preventing people from getting the swine flu or other types of influenza. The H1N1 virus is very contagious. It can be spread through close contact before people develop obvious symptoms, like a runny nose or a cough. There are some commonsense tips, though, to minimize the chance of catching or spreading H1N1.

PRACTICE GOOD HYGIENE FOR PREVENTION

Wash your hands! One of the most important ways to decrease the chance of catching or spreading H1N1 and other viruses is frequent hand washing. This should be done with traditional soap and water or with hand sanitizer gels that have been shown to kill viruses. Influenza viruses can live on surfaces for some time. The viruses spread when people touch things that infected people have touched. For example,

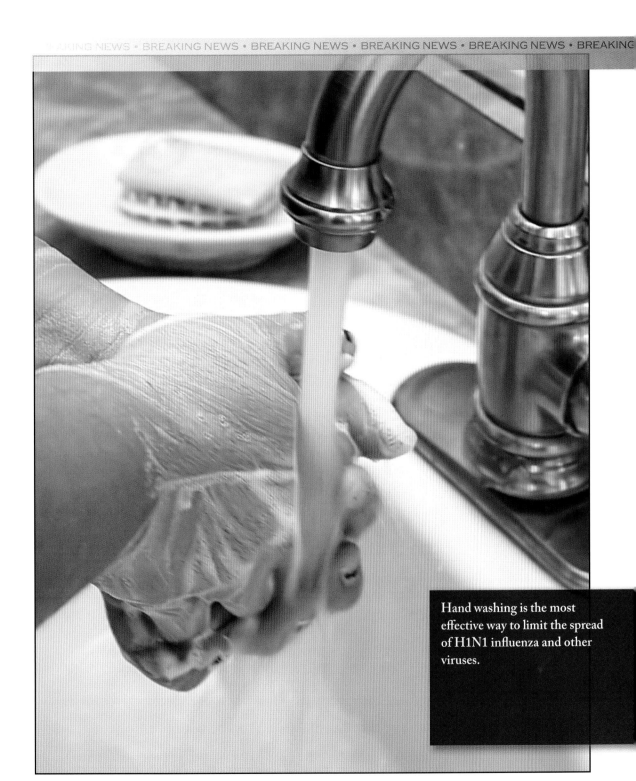

Hand washing is the most effective way to limit the spread of H1N1 influenza and other viruses.

it is a good idea to wash one's hands immediately after getting off of a public bus, train, or airplane. Many people travel every day by mass transit, and it is impossible to know which people on a bus or train have been sick. Of course, people should wash their hands whenever they sneeze or cough, too.

Another commonsense tip is learning how to sneeze properly. This may sound like a strange idea. However, scientific studies have shown that sneezing into one's sleeve or elbow instead of one's hands decreases the spread of respiratory viruses. This is likely because people touch everything with their hands. After sneezing on the hands, a person can spread lingering virus particles by touching everyday items, like doorknobs, that others will touch. One should also avoid touching one's eyes, nose, and mouth when sick, since viruses like H1N1 can hang out in all of these places.

Similarly, it makes sense to avoid being around other people who are sick. The CDC recommends that anyone who has symptoms of H1N1, like nasal congestion, cough, and fever, should stay home from school and work. This helps limit the contact of the sick person with healthy individuals so that the virus doesn't spread to more people. People also should not share toothbrushes, drinking glasses, or other utensils.

If you traveled on an airplane during the height of the H1N1 outbreak, you might have seen people wearing surgical face masks. This was a particularly popular thing to do in Japan, where hygiene and cleanliness are highly valued. For most people, though, wearing masks is not very effective, especially when they are worn for a long period of time. Although masks, when fitted properly, are good at limiting the spread of respiratory viruses like H1N1, most people do not get the masks to seal tightly on their faces. If there are gaps between the mask and the face, viruses can easily enter through these openings. Masks can also get damp after fifteen or twenty minutes due to moisture in the breath, causing them to break down. Then, they are much less effective at filtering and trapping virus particles.

The CDC advised in September 2009 that most people do not need to wear surgical masks in the community or in their homes, unless they are caring for someone with known H1N1 infection. Obviously, health care workers such as doctors and nurses should wear special face masks and other personal protective equipment, like gloves and gowns, when caring for patients with known or suspected H1N1 infection. Such protection limits the spread of H1N1 to these workers and to other patients.

VACCINATION

Get vaccinated! Although it is not fun to get a shot, getting the H1N1 vaccine and the regular flu vaccine is important. According to the CDC's Key Facts update in February 2010, "The flu vaccine is the single best way to protect against influenza illness." The Public Health Agency of Canada agreed strongly with this message. It is important to know that the seasonal flu vaccine does not protect people against the H1N1 strain. People have to get both vaccines. The seasonal flu vaccine is typically made up of two types of influenza A viruses and one type of influenza B virus that were commonly detected the prior year. For the 2009–2010 season, the vaccine contained an H3N2-like strain and an H1N1-like strain, which was different from the pandemic strain. It also contained an influenza B strain.

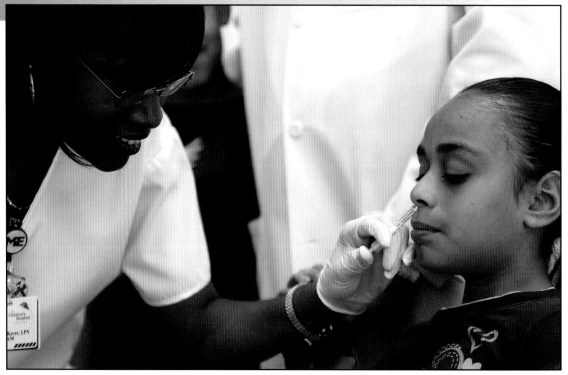

A child in New York City receives a dose of the intranasal H1N1 vaccine. The vaccine currently comes in two forms: a liquid given through the nose and a shot injected into the muscle.

How the Vaccine Works

To make the H1N1 vaccine, small bits of influenza viruses are processed to prevent them from being able to create a real infection when given to people. In 2009, there were two methods of processing H1N1 particles to make vaccines. One vaccine used inactivated (killed) H1N1 and was given as a regular injection into the muscle. The second vaccine was a nasal spray made from live, attenuated (weakened) H1N1. Both vaccines worked by stimulating the immune system to make protective antibodies against H1N1.

WHEN TO SEEK MEDICAL ATTENTION

Most people with H1N1 get through their illness without needing to be hospitalized. Anyone with severe symptoms of H1N1, though, should see a doctor for evaluation. It can be difficult to know if a person's symptoms are related to H1N1 or just the common cold, but it is better to be safe. If a person has extreme breathing difficulty, seems excessively sleepy, has extreme vomiting, or gets very dehydrated, he or she should be immediately seen by his or her doctor or evaluated in an emergency room. Symptoms and signs of H1N1 can come on or change very quickly. Unfortunately, some people, including some individuals who were otherwise young and healthy, have died because they did not seek or obtain proper medical attention in time.

Antibodies are special proteins that fight foreign substances in the body. They are made by certain white blood cells called B cells. After vaccination, it usually takes a few weeks for the body to make enough antibodies. The antibodies then circulate in the bloodstream, where they are ready to attack if they are challenged by a foreign invader.

When a vaccinated person is exposed to H1N1, the body recognizes the virus and ramps up production of antibodies against H1N1. Because the body has made these antibodies before, it can make new ones quickly. These protective antibodies can decrease the severity of flu symptoms or may prevent a person from getting the swine flu at all.

Students in Japan wear face masks to try to limit the spread of H1N1 influenza.

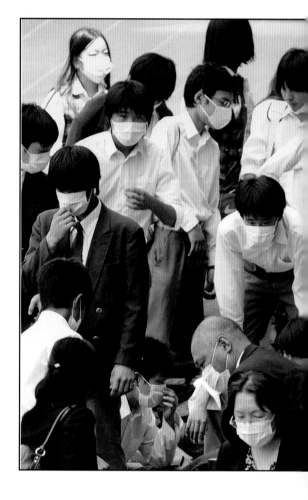

Side Effects

In rare cases, people can react negatively to vaccination. For example, anyone who has an allergy to eggs should not receive either the seasonal or H1N1 flu shots. The virus used in the current vaccines is grown in chicken eggs. Symptoms of a severe allergic reaction may include rash, throat swelling, or extreme difficulty breathing.

In rare cases, the seasonal and H1N1 flu shots have been linked to Guillain-Barré syndrome, a neurologic condition that involves muscle weakness. This condition usually gets better on its own without treatment, but some people have required hospitalization and died from it. Also, Guillain-Barré syndrome can last many weeks to months before it gets better. The syndrome is thought to have many different causes, not just influenza vaccinations.

In addition, certain groups of people should not get the live, attenuated intranasal vaccine. Even though the virus has been weakened, it

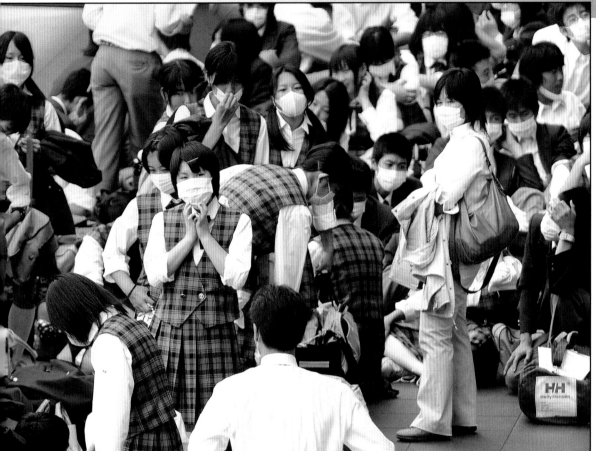

is still alive and has the potential to cause uncontrolled H1N1 infection in people whose immune systems do not work properly. The CDC's Advisory Council on Immunization Practices (ACIP) advised that people with chronic health problems, pregnant women, and children six months to two years only receive the inactivated flu shot, not the intranasal vaccine, due to their relatively weak immune systems.

People should discuss their medical concerns and ask questions about H1N1 vaccination in consultation with their health care providers. The CDC has published general guidelines regarding H1N1 vaccine safety, as well as helpful answers to frequently asked questions.

TREATMENT FOR H1N1

People with bad ear infections or bacterial pneumonias (lung infections) are often treated with antibiotics. For the most part, such infections usually get better once people complete a full course of antibiotic treatment. Are there medicines to treat H1N1, too?

Such medicines do indeed exist, although they don't actually kill the H1N1 virus. Treatment with antiviral medicines can decrease the length of time a person has flu symptoms, as well as the seriousness of these symptoms. Treatment is most effective when given within forty-eight hours of the start of flu symptoms. As a result, people with serious cases of H1N1 need to be evaluated very quickly by their health care providers. As discussed earlier, H1N1 was found to be universally resistant to some antiviral medications. Only oseltamivir (Tamiflu) and zanamivir (Relenza) were found to be effective against the 2009 H1N1 strain.

According to the instructions of major government agencies during the pandemic, antiviral medicines were only to be prescribed to people with very serious H1N1 infections. It was not deemed medically necessary to give these medicines to everyone with milder symptoms of the swine flu. If the medicines had been prescribed to everyone, it would have resulted in a worldwide shortage of effective antiviral medicines for patients who truly needed them.

CHAPTER 5

THE FUTURE OF SWINE FLU

H1N1 had been detected in more than two hundred countries by January 2010. Despite its widespread effects and much hype, the H1N1 pandemic of 2009 was probably the least deadly influenza pandemic in recent history. Although the strain had been unusually virulent and severe vaccine shortages had occurred, H1N1 ultimately resulted in fewer deaths than did the Spanish, Asian, and Hong Kong flu pandemics.

JUST ANOTHER PANDEMIC

Public health experts credit the H1N1 vaccine for slowing down the rapid spread and lethality of the H1N1 virus. Despite the delays in the vaccine's development, it was very effective in protecting people from the swine flu.

Media coverage throughout the United States and Canada was excellent in raising awareness about H1N1 and encouraging people to get vaccinated. Dr. Thomas Frieden, director of the CDC, noted that more than sixty million Americans had received the H1N1 vaccine by the beginning of 2010. CDC officials praised the media coverage of the H1N1 pandemic. They also pointed to the quick debunking of rumors through frequent public updates by the Obama administration,

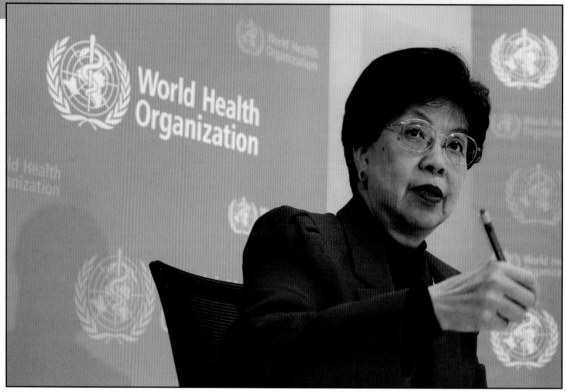

Margaret Chan, director-general of the World Health Organization, discusses the H1N1 pandemic at a press conference in Geneva, Switzerland.

the CDC, and the WHO. At the peak of the pandemic, these organizations held news conferences and educational seminars several times per week to educate the public about H1N1. The CDC created a special section on its Web site dedicated to current information about the H1N1 virus, including health tips, disease statistics, and vaccination updates. The HHS used its Web site http://www.flu.gov to keep people up-to-date on H1N1 and seasonal flu viruses.

What is the most current information? According to Frieden in a national press conference in December 2009, "We have an ebbing second wave [of H1N1 influenza], but an uncertain future." For now, people will just have to stay tuned to see what happens with H1N1.

SPEEDING THE VACCINE

The major issue with the H1N1 vaccine was its delay in production. This was largely due to the virus growing more slowly than anticipated. To make the vaccine, companies grew the H1N1 virus in chicken eggs. (Viruses cannot grow on their own, but have to live inside cells to be able to reproduce.) A protein called albumin, which is found inside chicken eggs, supported the growth of the virus. This traditional method of making vaccine has been used for decades. The method is a good way to mass-produce enough of the virus to make millions of vaccine doses, and it is how the seasonal flu vaccine is made.

While the method is generally effective, it can be time-consuming. Several pharmaceutical companies are investigating alternative, faster ways of making the vaccine that do not involve using chicken eggs. They are trying to make the vaccine using animal cell cultures instead of eggs. For instance, Novartis began to investigate a cell culture–based strategy in June 2009. This method did not involve as many specific steps and could be more automated, or accomplished by machines. As a result, it allowed more H1N1 virus to be produced in a shorter time frame. Novartis quickly developed this technology for more rapid production of the H1N1 vaccine. Health officials approved it for use in Germany in November 2009.

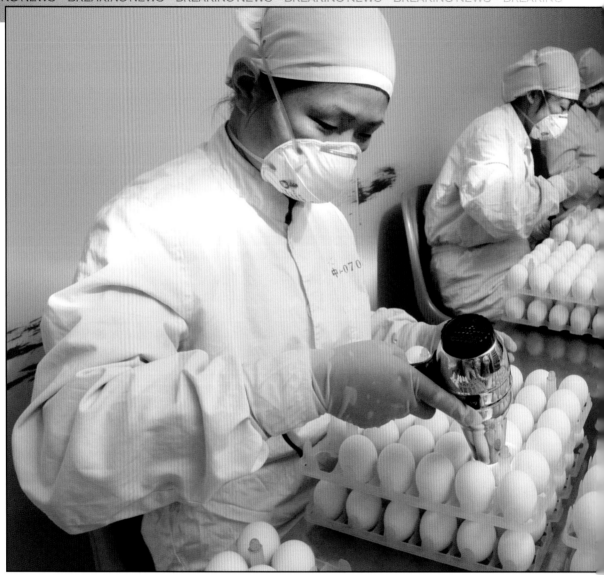

Shortly thereafter, other European countries approved similar cell culture–based vaccines. In the future, pharmaceutical companies and research laboratories will continue these and other approaches to vaccine development in an effort to improve both the quantity and the

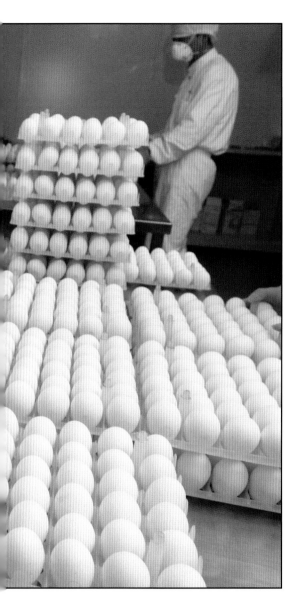

Millions of doses of H1N1 influenza vaccine were made by growing the virus in chicken eggs.

quality of the H1N1 vaccine. Using alternative approaches may also allow people who are allergic to eggs to be given the H1N1 vaccine safely.

H1N1's Impact on Travel, Now and in the Future

How has H1N1 affected national and international travel, and will there be more precautions in the future? As of early 2010, the WHO stated that it was safe to travel and that restrictions due to H1N1 concerns were not necessary. According to the organization, since the H1N1 virus has already spread throughout the world, there is no scientific reason to restrict people's travels in the hope of minimizing its spread. H1N1 is already just about everywhere. The organization did recommend that people refrain from traveling if

VACCINE RECALLS

In addition to problems with vaccine shortages and delays in production, the quality of some of the vaccine remains in question. In late 2009 and early 2010, millions of H1N1 vaccine doses were recalled. They were not pulled because of safety concerns, but because they were not as strong as they should have been when retested over time. However, the U.S. Food and Drug Administration (FDA) noted that people who received vaccines from the recalled batches did not need to be revaccinated. The vaccines were only slightly less powerful than they should have been and were probably effective at stimulating protective antibody production. As more vaccine doses are produced, pharmaceutical companies and government agencies will need to continue checking the vaccines for their safety and efficacy.

they feel ill and that they seek medical attention if they feel ill away from home.

In addition, the WHO did not call for passengers to be screened at airports to monitor flu symptoms. Decisions about whether to do this were primarily left to individual countries under the International Health Regulations of 2005. Nonetheless, many countries instituted quarantines in 2009 for North American travel and travelers. The Public Health Agency of Canada advised Canadians against nonessential travel to dozens of countries in Africa, South America, the Middle East, and Asia. These warnings were still in effect in the spring of 2010.

It seems likely that people will continue to be nervous about international travel, no matter what the official WHO recommendations are. Because it is so easy to spread viruses like H1N1 on a crowded airplane or train, taking personal responsibility for their health is one of the most important things that travelers can do.

THE EVER-CHANGING VIRUS

Even though the H1N1 virus was under better control by the spring of 2010, the future of the swine flu remains uncertain. It is not known if H1N1 can be eradicated (completely eliminated) or if it will continue to cause problems. Viruses and other infectious agents have the ability to mutate, or change their genes. These changes can have serious consequences. For instance, some mutations might make a virus more powerful, while others might make the virus resistant to medication.

During the peak of the H1N1 pandemic, mutations were already being detected in strains of H1N1 in several patients in Norway. These mutations may have made certain H1N1 viruses even deadlier: two Norwegian patients who had the mutated form of H1N1 died from severe infections. The Norwegian Institute of Public Health thought the mutation might have allowed the virus to enter more deeply into the respiratory tract, causing pneumonia. Other mutant strains of H1N1, which were resistant to the antiviral medication oseltamivir, were detected at a summer camp in North Carolina, as well as in Wales in the United Kingdom. Will the virus continue to mutate? It seems likely that it will, but the effects of such changes are currently unknown.

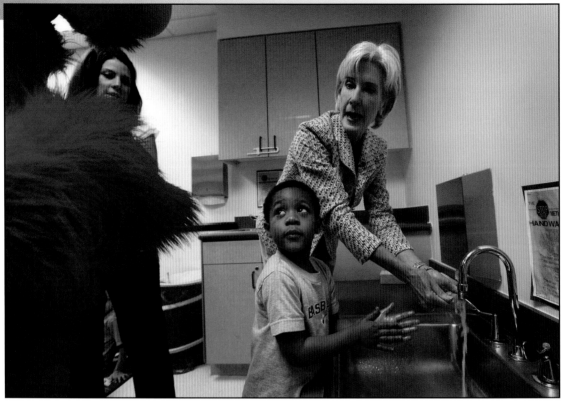

Kathleen Sebelius, the secretary of the Department of Health and Human Services, teaches children how to wash their hands properly to prevent the spread of H1N1.

There are two very good weapons against swine flu, thanks to modern medicine: vaccines to prevent or minimize H1N1 infection and antiviral medications to treat severe infections. Still, people must remain informed and alert. Taking protective measures, such as practicing good hygiene, is essential. People must also use common sense and stay home when they are sick. Infection with H1N1 and other influenza viruses causes serious illness and death throughout the world. Our mobile and global society makes it easy for such infections to spread quickly.

H1N1 has been detected in hundreds of countries. The pandemic has proved particularly devastating in countries with limited health care resources. Without proper medical facilities to care for severely ill patients, a large enough supply of antiviral medications, or sufficient vaccine doses, underdeveloped countries have seen a particularly high death toll from H1N1. No one knows what will happen next with the H1N1 virus. Will it continue its rampage of infection throughout the world? How many more people will be affected? Will the H1N1 virus mutate and become even stronger? Will it remain treatable with antiviral medications? Or will the swine flu eventually disappear? Only time will tell.

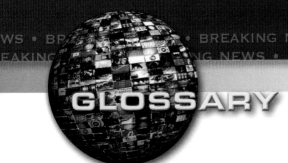

GLOSSARY

aerosol A suspension of fine solid or liquid particles in a gas.

antibody A protein that acts against infectious agents. Antibodies are made by special white blood cells called B cells; production of antibodies is stimulated by vaccination.

chronic Long-lasting; constant.

complacent Not concerned; self-satisfied.

contact A coming together or touching, as of objects or surfaces.

epidemic An outbreak of contagious disease that spreads rapidly among the people in an area or population.

eradicate To eliminate, remove, or destroy.

hemagglutinin A protein that causes cells to stick together. In the case of H1N1, hemagglutinin allows the influenza virus to attach to host cells.

hygiene Cleanliness.

mutate To undergo a change in the genetic material (DNA or RNA).

neuraminidase A protein on the surface of infectious agents that breaks down sugars. In the case of H1N1, neuraminidase allows the influenza virus to enter host cells.

pandemic An epidemic that occurs over a large geographic area or even worldwide.

potent Strong; powerful.

resistant Not treatable; not responsive to medication.

respiratory Related to breathing or the lungs.

strain A variety, especially of microorganisms.

susceptible Easily affected; vulnerable to the effects of.

symptom An indicator of disease.

transmit To spread.

vaccine A preparation of an infectious agent that is used to provide immunity to a disease by causing the body to produce antibodies.

virus An infectious agent made of nucleic acid (DNA or RNA) and proteins that must reside within cells to reproduce.

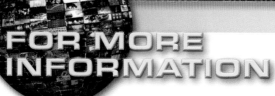

Centers for Disease Control and Prevention (CDC)

1600 Clifton Road

Atlanta, GA 30333

(800) CDC-INFO [232-4636]

Web site: http://www.cdc.gov

The CDC is one of the major divisions of the U.S. Department of Health and Human Services. Its mission is to provide the expertise, information, and tools that people and communities need to protect health. Areas of focus include health promotion; prevention of disease, injury, and disability; and preparedness for new health threats.

Health Canada

A.L. 0900C2

Ottawa, ON K1A 0K9

Canada

(866) 225-0709

Web site: http://www.hc-sc.gc.ca

Health Canada is the federal department that helps Canadians to maintain and improve their health, while respecting individual choices and circumstances.

Public Health Agency of Canada

130 Colonnade Road

A.L. 6501H

Ottawa, ON K1A 0K9

Canada

(613) 957-2991

Web site: http://www.phac-aspc.gc.ca

The Public Health Agency of Canada's primary goal is to protect and
improve the health of Canadians and help reduce pressures on the
health care system.

U.S. Department of Health and Human Services (HHS)

200 Independence Avenue SW

Washington, DC 20201

(877) 696-6775

Web site: http://www.hhs.gov

The HHS is the U.S. government's principal agency for protecting the
health of Americans and providing essential human services. For
more information about influenza, see the agency's special Web site
Flu.gov. It provides comprehensive information on seasonal, swine,
bird, and pandemic flu for health and emergency preparedness
professionals, policy makers, government and business leaders, and
the general public.

U.S. Food and Drug Administration (FDA)

10903 New Hampshire Avenue

Silver Spring, MD 20993-0002

(888) INFO-FDA [463-6332]

Web site: http://www.fda.gov

The FDA, an agency of the U.S. Department of Health and Human Services, protects the public health by assuring the safety, efficacy, and security of drugs, biological products, medical devices, foods, cosmetics, and other products. It advances the public health by supporting innovations that make medicines and foods more effective, safer, and more affordable. It also educates the public about using medicines and foods to improve health.

World Health Organization (WHO)
Avenue Appia 20
1211 Geneva 27
Switzerland
+ 41 22 791 21 11
Web site: http://www.who.int/en
The WHO is the directing and coordinating authority for health within the United Nations system. It is responsible for providing leadership on global health matters, shaping the health research agenda, setting standards, articulating evidence-based policy options, providing technical support to countries, and monitoring and assessing health trends.

Web Sites

Due to the changing nature of Internet links, Rosen Publishing has developed an online list of Web sites related to the subject of this book. This site is updated regularly. Please use this link to access the list:

http://www.rosenlinks.com/hls/sflu

Burgan, Michael. *Developing Flu Vaccines* (Science Missions). Chicago, IL: Raintree, 2011.

Chilman-Blair, Kim. *Medikidz Explain Swine Flu* (Superheroes on a Medical Mission). New York, NY: Rosen Publishing Group, 2011.

Devlin, Roni K. *Influenza* (Biographies of Disease). Westport, CT: Greenwood Press, 2008.

Dorrance, John M. *Global Time Bomb: Surviving the H1N1 Swine Flu Pandemic and Other Global Health Threats*. Seattle, WA: Pacific Publishing Studio, 2009.

Drexler, Madeline. *Emerging Epidemics: The Menace of New Infections*. New York, NY: Penguin Books, 2010.

Dumar, A. M. *Swine Flu: What You Need to Know*. Brooklyn, NY: Brownstone Books, 2009.

Goldsmith, Connie. *Influenza* (USA Today Health Reports: Diseases and Disorders). Minneapolis, MN: Twenty-First Century Books, 2011.

Grady, Denise. *Deadly Invaders: Virus Outbreaks Around the World, from Marburg Fever to Avian Flu*. Boston, MA: Kingfisher, 2006.

Hoffmann, Gretchen. *The Flu* (Health Alert). New York, NY: Marshall Cavendish Benchmark, 2007.

Kelly, Evelyn B. *Investigating Influenza and Bird Flu: Real Facts for Real Lives* (Investigating Diseases). Berkeley Heights, NJ: Enslow Publishers, 2010.

Kolata, Gina Bari. *Flu: The Story of the Great Influenza Pandemic of 1918 and the Search for the Virus That Caused It*. New York, NY: Touchstone, 2005.

Krohn, Katherine E. *The 1918 Flu Pandemic* (Graphic Library). Mankato, MN: Capstone Press, 2008.

Kupperberg, Paul. *The Influenza Pandemic of 1918–1919* (Great Historic Disasters). New York, NY: Chelsea House, 2008.

Moore, Peter. *The Little Book of Pandemics: 50 of the World's Most Virulent Plagues and Infectious Diseases*. New York, NY: Collins, 2007.

Ollhoff, Jim. *The Flu*. Edina, MN: ABDO Publishing Company, 2010.

Parks, Peggy J. *Influenza* (Compact Research Series). San Diego, CA: ReferencePoint Press, 2011.

Ricks, Delthia. *100 Questions & Answers About Influenza*. Sudbury, MA: Jones and Bartlett, 2009.

Stephenson, Terence. *Swine Flu/H1N1: The Facts*. Philadelphia, PA: Jessica Kingsley, 2009.

Stille, Darlene R. *Outbreak! The Science of Pandemics*. Mankato, MN: Compass Point Books, 2011.

Youngerman, Barry. *Pandemics and Global Health* (Global Issues). New York, NY: Facts On File, 2008.

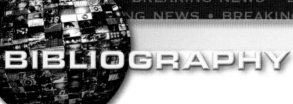

BIBLIOGRAPHY

Allday, Erin. "Distribution Plans Fall Short for H1N1 Vaccine."
SFGate.com, December 14, 2009. Retrieved June 22, 2010 (http://
articles.sfgate.com/2009-12-14/news/17224375_1_swine-flu-
vaccine-immunization-branch-high-risk).

Associated Press. "Amid Shortage, Big NYC Firms Get Swine
Vaccine." MSNBC.com, November 5, 2009. Retrieved June 22,
2010 (http://www.msnbc.msn.com/id/33655838/ns/health-
cold_and_flu).

Associated Press. "Public Concern Over H1N1 Waning, Poll
Finds: Just 40 Percent Worried About Getting Sick, Down
from 52 Percent." MSNBC.com, December 22, 2009. Retrieved
February 22, 2010 (http://www.msnbc.msn.com/id/34524874/ns/
health-cold_and_flu).

Burns, Judith. "Health Officials Frustrated by H1N1 Vaccine Shortage."
WSJ.com, November 4, 2009. Retrieved January 14, 2010 (http://
online.wsj.com/article/SB125735930128328447.html).

Centers for Disease Control and Prevention. "CDC Estimates of 2009
H1N1 Influenza Cases, Hospitalizations, and Deaths in the United
States, April 2009–January 16, 2010." 2010. Retrieved February 22,
2010 (http://www.cdc.gov/h1n1flu/estimates_2009_h1n1.htm).

Centers for Disease Control and Prevention. "Key Facts About 2009
H1N1 Flu Vaccine." March 8, 2010. Retrieved February 22, 2010
(http://www.cdc.gov/h1n1flu/vaccination/vaccine_keyfacts.htm).

Centers for Disease Control and Prevention. "CDC 2009 H1N1 Flu." 2009. Retrieved January 14, 2010 (http://www.cdc.gov/H1N1FLU).

Deprez, Esmé E. "Banks' H1N1 Flu Vaccines Stir Outrage." *BusinessWeek*, November 5, 2009. Retrieved June 22, 2010 (http://www.businessweek.com/bwdaily/dnflash/content/nov2009/db2009115_844446_page_2.htm).

Garrett, Laurie. "The Path of a Pandemic: How One Virus Spread from Pigs and Birds to Humans Around the Globe. And Why Microbes Like the H1N1 Flu Have Become a Growing Threat." *Newsweek*, May 11, 2009. Retrieved January 14, 2010 (http://www.newsweek.com/id/195692).

Harvard School of Public Health. "Nearly Half of Americans Believe H1N1 Outbreak Is Over, Poll Finds." February 5, 2010. Retrieved February 22, 2010 (http://www.hsph.harvard.edu/news/press-releases/2010-releases/poll-half-of-americans-believe-h1n1-outbreak-over.html).

Knox, Richard. "Swine Flu Vaccine Shortage: Why?" NPR.org, October 26, 2009. Retrieved January 14, 20710 (http://www.npr.org/templates/story/story.php?storyId=114156775).

Landau, Elizabeth. "To Vaccinate or Not? Some Wary on H1N1 Choice." CNN.com, October 9, 2009. Retrieved January 14, 2010 (http://www.cnn.com/2009/HEALTH/10/09/h1n1.vaccine.skepticism).

McNeil, Donald G., Jr. "U.S. Reaction to Swine Flu: Apt and Lucky." *New York Times*, January 1, 2010. Retrieved February 22, 2010 (http://www.nytimes.com/2010/01/02/health/02flu.html).

New York Academy of Sciences. "Human Swine Flu (H1N1) and Novel Influenza Pandemics." 2009. Retrieved January 14, 2010 (http://www.nyas.org/Publications/EBriefings/Detail. aspx?cid=d48b4f6e-74a0-4cd8-a0eb-8c831c020d78#).

Public Health Agency of Canada. "Frequently Asked Questions About H1N1." 2010. Retrieved February 22, 2010 (http://www. phac-aspc.gc.ca/alert-alerte/h1n1/faq/faq_rg_h1n1-fvv-eng.php).

Ruiz, Rebecca. "Behind the H1N1 Vaccine Shortage." Forbes.com, October 30, 2009. Retrieved June 22, 2010 (http://www.forbes.com/ 2009/10/27/swine-flu-vaccine-lifestyle-health-h1n1-shortage.html).

Shear, Michael D., and Rob Stein. "Why Is There Such a Shortage of H1N1 Vaccine?" *Washington Post*, October 27, 2009. Retrieved January 14, 2010 (http://www.washingtonpost.com/wpdyn/ content/article/2009/10/26/AR2009102603487.html).

University of California–Los Angeles. "H1N1 Virus Spreads Easily by Plane." ScienceDaily.com, January 8, 2010. Retrieved February 22, 2010 (http://www.sciencedaily.com/ releases/2010/01/100107114724.htm).

Walsh, Bryan. "Swine Flu: 5 Things You Need to Know About the Outbreak." Time.com, April 27, 2009. Retrieved January 14, 2010 (http://www.time.com/time/health/article/ 0,8599,1894029,00.html).

World Health Organization: Regional Office for the Western Pacific. "Overview of the Current Pandemic H1N1 2009 Situation." 2009. Retrieved January 14, 2010 (http://www.wpro.who.int/ health_topics/h1n1).

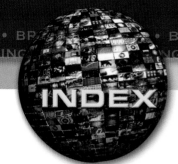

INDEX

ABOUT THE AUTHOR

Sarah K. Tasian, MD, is a pediatric hematologist-oncologist at the University of California, San Francisco (UCSF), where she performs laboratory research in pediatric leukemia and takes care of children with various blood disorders and cancers. She graduated summa cum laude from the University of Notre Dame and Alpha Omega Alpha from the Baylor College of Medicine. She trained in pediatrics at the University of Washington/Seattle Children's Hospital and in pediatric hematology-oncology at UCSF. She has a particular interest in infections in immunocompromised patients and has published a scientific article about the complications of influenza in children with cancer. Dr. Tasian lives in San Francisco with her husband and young son.

PHOTO CREDITS

Cover Joe Raedle/Getty Images; pp. 4–5 Hemera/Thinkstock; p. 8 Pasieka/Photo Researchers, Inc.; p. 11 Luis Acosta/AFP/Getty Images; p. 15 Archive Photos/Getty Images; p. 17 AFP/Getty Images; p. 19 CDC/James Gathany; pp. 22–23, 26 George Frey/Getty Images; pp. 30–31 The White House/Getty Images; p. 32 Nicholas Kamm/AFP/Getty Images; p.35 Shutterstock.com; p. 38 Mario Tama/Getty Images; pp. 40–41 Kazuhiro Nogi/AFP/Getty Images; p. 44 Fabrice Coffrini/AFP/Getty Images; pp. 46–47 Newscom; p. 50 Robert Giroux/Getty Images; interior graphics © www.istockphoto.com/Chad Anderson (globe) © www.istockphoto.com/ymgerman (map) © www.istockphoto.com/Brett Lamb (satellite dish).

Editor: Andrea Sclarow; Photo Researcher: Peter Tomlinson